Coumadin

An easy to follow guide from a patient's perspective

Cath Atkin

ISBN: 978-0-9933499-0-4

Published by Catkin Publishing

www.eatonwarfarin.com

Disclaimer

This book is not designed, or intended, to provide you with medical advice, professional diagnosis, opinion, treatment or services. This book is not intended as a substitute for the medical advice of doctors or other medical or healthcare professionals. You should regularly consult a doctor (or other relevant medical professional) in matters relating to your health. You should not use the information in this book as a substitute for a consultation with a doctor or other medical professional.

Although the author has made every effort to ensure that the information in this book was correct at the time of publication, the author and the publisher do not assume and hereby disclaim any liability to any party for any loss, damage, or disruption caused by errors or omissions, whether such errors or omissions result from negligence, accident, or any other cause. The author is not liable or responsible for any advice, course of treatment, diagnosis or any other information or services you obtain or follow as a result of reading this book.

IF YOU BELIEVE YOU HAVE A MEDICAL EMERGENCY, YOU SHOULD IMMEDIATELY CALL THE RELEVANT EMERGENCY SERVICES IN YOUR JURISDICTION. If you believe you have any other health problem, or if you have any questions regarding your health, you should promptly consult your doctor (or other relevant healthcare professionals). Never disregard medical or professional advice, or delay seeking it on account of something you read in this book. Do not rely on information in this book instead of seeking professional medical advice. You should also ask your physician, or other healthcare professionals, to assist you in interpreting the information in this book or in applying this information to your individual case.

Medical information changes constantly. Therefore the information in this book should not be considered current, complete or exhaustive, nor should you rely on such information to recommend a course of treatment for you or any other individual.

Acknowledgements

I want to thank a number of people for different aspects of the support they have given me to help my recovery and also in writing this book. Now that I am back to full health I am able to give thanks from the bottom of my heart.

To my Mum, Eleanor and Great Aunt, Nan, who have always believed in me and been there whenever I needed them. Always showing kindness and providing words of wisdom when I required it. Mum, it's with thanks to you and Dad for raising me to have such a positive attitude, a strong resilience and to believe that anything is possible. Without this I would have certainly struggled on my road to recovery never mind looking at how I can help others in sharing everything I have learned. I am grateful more than you will ever know.

To my friends Sarah Richardson, Demi Powell, Helen Geddes, Lisa Ames-White and Suzzy Grant who have been there throughout this, putting up with my struggles and encouraging me to get back on my feet, from dragging me out for coffees to dealing with the doctors. Your patience has been a virtue and your support has been so very much appreciated. Thanks ladies.

To my friends Katrina and Jim Gracie, who have helped me out in so many areas, helping me with so many things including taking on Zeus when I needed and advice when required. Nothing has ever been a problem to you, thank you for always being there.

To Laura Draper, who has come in to work with me and hit the ground running. Laura has worked tirelessly with me to pull this book and website together. I am extremely grateful for your diligence and patience Laura and without these strong traits of yours and the amount of time you spent on it, this would have been a very different book.

There are so many people who have been involved in some way from helping me to get back on my feet again and bring this information to print. I am eternally grateful to you all and appreciate every single thing that has been offered. I have been blessed not only to have been through such a journey to get back to full recovery but also to have such amazing and wonderful people around me.

CONTENTS

For further information and resources
visit
www.eatonwarfarin.com

Introduction

With all the amazing access to data we have in today's digital world, why is it still so difficult to find simple, easy to understand information on one of the world's most widely used medications?

Coumadin®, which is also known generically as warfarin, is a widely used *anticoagulant* drug often referred to as a *'blood thinner'.*

Through this book, I aim to present information about Coumadin from the perspective of someone who is taking this medication. I have tried to provide a simple explanation of how the drug works, its main purposes and benefits, and relate this to what being on this medication has meant for me. We are all different so please be aware that a lot of the material contained in this book relates specifically to how Coumadin has affected me. There are other books available that offer a more detailed explanation of Coumadin from a medical perspective. My aim, however, has been to provide a straightforward guide that gives quick access to some of the important aspects of taking Coumadin for anyone who has been prescribed this drug. I hope other Coumadin users will find this useful.

About the Author

Until recently, I did not have any experience of **'blood thinners'** *such as Coumadin, nor did I know anyone who took them. I had always assumed these were drugs prescribed to* **older people** *but how wrong I was. In my early 40's, when I was running my own business, I would often become very tired but generally put this down to exhaustion from working too much. Later, I began to get* ***migraines*** *for the first time in my life but again put it down to stress and carried on. The migraines caused me to feel a* **sharp pain** *in my* **left eye***; sometimes I would* **lose part of my vision** *for perhaps a minute or so. Only later did I realize that these migraines had been an* ***early warning sign*** *of what was to come. My life then changed quite dramatically when I had the opportunity to sell my business – no more stress! The frequency of the migraines reduced but the tiredness never really got any better. A year later while on holiday in Europe, and completely out of the blue, I suffered a stroke while taking a shower. At first I thought I had tweaked a nerve in my neck because I* ***nearly fainted*** *and* ***lost the feeling in my arm*** *but as my condition worsened I was rushed to hospital. The doctors told me I had experienced an* ***acute ischemic attack*** *- a blood clot in the brain to you and me!*

I always thought strokes affected older people, not someone my age.

While in hospital, I was given **'baby aspirin'** *or* **Plavix®** *(75mg aspirin). I was also given a* **statin** *called* simvastatin; *the dosage was 10mg daily. These were given to me to reduce my risk of having another stroke. What had caused the stroke was unclear. I had been a smoker for 14 years, (not good but the doctors felt this was unlikely to have caused a stroke), I was no longer in a stressful job, my blood pressure was normal, and although my cholesterol was on the high side of the recommended range this should not have been enough to contribute to the stroke. None of it made any sense so, once I returned home, I had to undergo a lot more tests to try and get to the root cause.*

After further investigation I was diagnosed with a blood clotting disorder called antiphospholipid syndrome **(APS)***. This diagnosis suddenly made sense of so many of the other symptoms which had been troubling me - like the tiredness and migraines. APS, sometimes referred to as* **'sticky blood'***, is also known as* **Hughes syndrome** *– named after* Professor Graham Hughes, *who discovered the illness. He is still practicing today and I have been fortunate enough to be treated by one of his colleagues at* London Bridge Hospital - Professor Munther Khamashta.

For more information and links relating to Hughes syndrome or APS visit
www.eatonwarfarin.com

My initial diagnosis of ***APS****, however, was made by a hematologist at my local hospital who put me on* ***Coumadin*** *immediately. I was very fortunate to have been correctly diagnosed quickly. Looking through the forums on 'sticky blood' disorder I discovered that so many people are misdiagnosed or suffer for years prior to receiving a correct diagnosis and being treated with an anticoagulant drug.*

For me, being diagnosed and put on Coumadin within a short space of time was a ***positive thing****. I was happy to take Coumadin to help prevent me becoming ill again. Having had such a hard time recovering from my stroke I was glad of anything that would reduce the risk of me having another. I was therefore surprised by the frequent negative reactions I came across when I told people I was taking Coumadin. I lost count of the number of times I heard comments such as,* ***'Coumadin? I wouldn't touch that!', 'it's a killer drug' or 'that's rat poison'.*** *Although these comments made me feel upset and confused they also made me realize how little people know about the drug. I felt it was really important that anyone coming in contact with Coumadin – those prescribed the drug, their carer's, friends or family – should have simple and clear information available to them. Understanding more fully about the benefits and potential dangers of taking Coumadin has helped me to accept my treatment as an important part of my daily routine.*

Yes, Coumadin can kill. If not managed effectively it can cause major bleeding. The important thing is to learn how to manage it safely.

And so this brings me to where I am today. My aim is to promote better understanding of Coumadin, and its management, and to provide straightforward and easily accessible resources to help others.

When dealing with medical issues it is normal to include a disclaimer which states: 'always seek the opinion of your doctor' as at the beginning of this book.

HOWEVER ...

I want to reinforce the message that when taking Coumadin, you MUST speak to your doctor about any changes you plan to make. Coumadin seems to interact both positively and negatively with almost everything. What we eat, other medication, dietary supplements, hydration levels and our individual physiology each have an effect on how Coumadin works. Therefore any changes, no matter how small, can alter the effect Coumadin has on you and can be dangerous! So avoid thinking: 'I don't want to bother the doctor', or 'I don't have time'. Consult your doctor before making changes to your diet or trying anything new such as supplements. Be aware there can be dangerous side effects associated with change which could place your health at serious risk.

Please also remember that I write from a personal point of view and in doing so, I have illustrated the challenges I had in starting and managing Coumadin. I am not offering medical advice.

CHAPTER 1

Why is Coumadin prescribed?

Coumadin is commonly used in the treatment of individuals who have suffered, or are at risk of having, a **heart attack, stroke, pulmonary embolism (PE)** or **deep vein thrombosis (DVT)**.

In general, the above *health events* are the result of an **unwanted blood clot**. I use the term 'unwanted' because we all want our blood to clot at certain times, such as when we have a cut, so that the bleeding will stop. For some of us, however, not only does our blood clot outside the body as it should do, but it also has a tendency to form clots inside the body with potentially catastrophic results.

An unwanted clot could begin to **form** anywhere **in the bloodstream**. Some clots will stay where they have formed while others will **break away** and travel through the blood vessels. A travelling clot can come to rest if it reaches a blood vessel that is **too narrow** or gets caught on some **fatty deposits**. The real problems start if the clot forms, or come to rest, at a main organ and blood flow is reduced. The most common health events caused by clots are,

- **heart attack** – when a clot obstructs blood flow to the heart
- **stroke** – when a clot obstructs blood flow to the head

- **pulmonary embolism** – when a clot obstructs blood flow to the lungs
- **dvt** – clot in the leg at high risk of breaking off and travelling to a main organ

Coumadin is one of a number of medications that can be prescribed to **help prevent blood clots forming.** Most people who are prescribed Coumadin will have health conditions requiring *ongoing use of the drug*. However, Coumadin is also used for people who are at **short term risk of blood clots**, for example, after surgery.

The majority of people in the US requiring anticoagulant treatment are prescribed Coumadin. If you don't react well to Coumadin, or your condition is better suited to one of the alternatives, another anticoagulant may be recommended.

Shortly after suffering my stroke I was diagnosed with ***antiphospholipid syndrome (APS).*** *This is an auto immune disorder which makes my blood clot* *more easily than that of the average person, putting me at risk of many serious health conditions including heart attack, stroke, DVT and pulmonary embolism. Having APS means that I will* ***always be at risk*** *of developing blood clots so it is vital for me to be prescribed a medicine which will help towards preventing this. I was told that Coumadin was the most suitable medication for my condition and, fortunately, it works well for me.*

CHAPTER 2

How does Coumadin work?

We have seen that **Coumadin** is prescribed to help prevent clots forming in the blood which could lead to a stroke, heart attack or other serious health condition.

I am not going to attempt to explain every aspect of how Coumadin controls the formation of blood clots – there are plenty of medical books available for that!

Put simply, blood is supposed to clot so that bleeding stops after an injury – this is called **coagulation**.

Coagulation is controlled by a group of **proteins** made in the liver called **clotting factors**. These clotting factors **need a supply of** Vitamin K **to operate**.

In basic terms, Coumadin works by doing two jobs,

1. Reducing the production of the **clotting factors**
2. Limiting the availability of **Vitamin K**

and, **as a result, it takes longer for the blood to clot** and unwanted blood clots are less likely to form.

It is likely that you will come across people referring to Coumadin as a 'blood thinner'. This is not technically correct as Coumadin is not actually thinning your blood, just making it less susceptible to clotting.

When I was first prescribed Coumadin, I tried to find out more about what it was and how it worked. Anyone who has been prescribed Coumadin, particularly those who have had a stroke, will appreciate that there is not a lot of easily accessible information on the drug and that the material that is available is ***not easy to understand****. As my cognitive processing was affected by the stroke, I struggled to make sense of the data I could find. Most of the information was very technical and I lacked the energy to decipher it because performing basic tasks took most of my energy at this time. I quickly realized that the type of easy to understand information that I was looking for was not out there. There and then I decided that, as soon as I was able, I would set about providing other Coumadin users with the sort of* ***basic manual*** *I had hoped to find when I first wanted information.*

CHAPTER 3

Starting Coumadin Therapy

Once a doctor, or other medical professional, has decided that you need to start Coumadin therapy their main aim is to find <u>the correct level of Coumadin for you</u> as quickly as possible.

Some medical practitioners prefer to start by giving **heparin injections** as this quickly **regulates the clotting of the blood** while the required level of Coumadin is building up. Heparin is another type of anti-coagulant which works in a different way to Coumadin to prevent blood clots forming.

When I started Coumadin therapy, I was also given daily Fragmin® (a type of heparin) injections in my stomach. I was told this was a 'belt and braces' approach, which would further <u>reduce the possibility of clots</u> during the <u>initial phase</u> of Coumadin therapy. The injections stopped when my Coumadin levels were near the desired range.

It is important that heparin injections are stopped, or reduced, as the <u>desired range</u> or **Therapeutic Range** of Coumadin is approached. Your doctor will be trying to establish a level that will slow down the clotting of your blood but care must be taken not to take this too far the other way as this could cause a *<u>hemorrhage</u>*. Excessive levels of Coumadin can cause **life-threatening bleeding** so its' use must be carefully regulated.

It is normal to start on a low dose of Coumadin and have this increased gradually. During this period **blood tests** will be done **frequently** to monitor the effect of the level of Coumadin on your blood clotting. When starting Coumadin it is likely that you will have blood tests on a daily basis with the frequency reducing as your levels start to come under control. This process can take anywhere between a few days and several weeks, depending on the individual. Remember, we are all different so the time it will take for each of us will vary.

*For me, it took over **6 weeks** to reach to the right level. I had blood tests every day during the **first week** and every second day during the **second week**. This was then reduced to blood tests twice a week and eventually once a week as I neared the desired range. During this initial period my doctor increased my dosage of Coumadin one mg at a time. When my correct level of Coumadin was reached the frequency of the blood tests was reduced to once every 6 weeks.*

CHAPTER 4

Managing your Coumadin dosage

Once the desired level of Coumadin is achieved changes can still occur which **may require increases**, or **decreases**, in the number of milligrams (mg)you take. Do not think that because you start off on a fixed number of mgs each day that it will always remain that way. Sometimes you may be required to take a *combination* of different doses over a number of days. There is also no point in comparing your dosage level with others. Some people will require to be on as little as 3mg daily, while others might take 17mg a day. The amount of Coumadin you take is not important. What matters is **maintaining the clotting rate** of your blood.

My normal dose has been 12mg per day. Recently, due to some changes, my dosage has been changed to 12/13/13. This means I follow a 3 day pattern of 12mg for one day, followed by two days at 13mg, then back to 12mg and so on.

One thing is certain: if you are on Coumadin for life, you will have *regular checks* with your doctor or anticoagulant specialist. It can be **challenging getting used to being on Coumadin** and having to undergo frequent testing. You will start to become aware that there are many factors that can alter your level of Coumadin and at times you will need to revert to more intensive periods of testing so that your doctor can maintain your correct range. The important thing is to try and be in tune with your body and **not to hesitate to seek medical advice** if you think things are not as they should be.

At first I found it quite hard being on a new drug and getting used to all the implications of being on Coumadin but now I do not mind the monthly or 6-weekly checks. As well as my regular checks, my doctors are happy for me to go in and have an <u>*additional blood test*</u> *if I do not feel quite right. I have had occasion to do this following a* ***change of diet*** *or when I have been on* ***painkillers*** *and have felt unwell. I am starting to be able to recognize if my levels of Coumadin are either too high, or too low, and know a visit to my doctor is required. The doctor can then reset my dose if necessary but I will* <u>***never self-dose***</u>.

You will be advised of the *correct time of day* to take your dosage of Coumadin by your doctor or anticoagulant specialist. In the US, Coumadin users are normally advised to <u>**take the medication at 5:00 p.m. every night**</u>. There are a number of reasons for this. Firstly, blood tests to check your Coumadin level are normally done in the morning. This allows time for the doctor to receive the test results and **advise you of any required changes to your dosage** before it is due that evening. Also, taking your dosage in the morning prior to a blood test will affect the blood test result.

It is important to **take your Coumadin every day as prescribed** and to always take it at the **same time of day**. If you do forget to take your dose at the correct time there are guidelines on the Coumadin package leaflet telling you what to do.

If you have **missed a dose** and are unsure what to do, contact your doctor or anticoagulation specialist, and check what the **right advice** is **for you**.

If you accidentally take an **extra dose** or take **too much** Coumadin, speak to your doctor, or emergency service for advice **straightaway**.

In the early days, I thought that it was critical that I received my test results, and any new dosage, on the same day that my blood test had been done. This was particularly difficult when my doctor's surgery was closed at the weekend and I was having to go to the hospital for the tests. The hospital were supposed to phone me with the results and I would start to panic if they did not contact me by the end of the day. On occasion, I even called the 'out-of-hours' service to ask them to obtain the results. I have since learned that, unless I feel very unwell or am bleeding, it is fine to obtain the results and dosage the next day. My doctor has instructed me to take my medication at 6pm every night and remembering this can be a challenge! I have been known to forget to take medication in the past so when I was prescribed Coumadin I ***set an alarm*** *on my* ***phone*** *and another on my UP by Jawbone* ***wristband*** *to remind me. Have I always taken the medication at 6pm on the dot?* ***No****, but as long as I have taken it within a couple of hours before or after 6pm I have not had any issues. I have never missed one of my daily doses of Coumadin completely so I can't share any personal experience of this.*

CHAPTER 5

Understanding Your Blood Testing

As discussed, the aim of your doctor, or anticoagulant specialist, is to get your levels of Coumadin within a desired range and then keep it there. The reason for taking Coumadin is to *reduce the clotting tendency* of the blood, not to stop it from clotting completely. This can be a bit of a fine balancing act. Your daily dose of Coumadin needs to be monitored, and adjusted if necessary, to keep this **'clotting time'** within a **target range**. This is achieved through regular testing.

Understanding the tests, and their results, can all be a **bit daunting at first**. At times it may seem like a whole new language! In this section I will go into a bit more detail about testing and try and explain some of the terms you are likely to come across.

How are the tests performed?

The most commonly used form of testing involves withdrawing **blood from a vein in the arm**. This blood sample is then sent to a laboratory to be analyzed. The results of the test will be sent back to the doctor, who can then contact his patient to discuss any **action** required, such as a **change to their Coumadin dose**.

These blood tests may take place at your doctor's surgery, hematology unit or hospital or be carried out by a medical professional at home.

Instead of taking a blood sample to send to the laboratory your nurse or doctor can use a **portable device** to carry out testing. This is commonly known as **'point of care'** testing. It is done on the spot and only requires a drop of blood which is taken from a **finger prick**. The device is similar to ones used to test blood sugar levels in diabetic patients and is usually able to present the results in a matter of minutes.

Another form of testing is **self-monitoring**. This involves the **patient** conducting the test **at home**. This option requires the patient to firstly undergo **thorough training**. Tests must be performed as often as the doctor advises and an appropriate lifestyle must be maintained. After performing the **self-check** the patient must **call in the results** to their doctor to discuss dosage. Very occasionally people using self-monitoring will also actually **self-dose**. Self-monitoring is not suitable for everyone and is an option that must be discussed at length with your doctor or coagulation specialist.

My testing is done by blood tests at the doctor's surgery. I was interested in the option of self-monitoring and ***discussed it*** *with my doctor; I was even willing to buy my own self-test machine. However, both my doctor and the hematologist advised against this. They explained that the training is extensive and the machines must be calibrated regularly at the hospital to ensure similar readings are given to that of a venous test. I was advised that it would be better for me to* ***continue with blood tests*** *at a doctor's surgery. While there would have been advantages to being able to self-test I feel happy that I receive regular checks by my doctor and that the dosing is undertaken by medical professionals.*

PT and INR

Two terms that you will come across over and over again, in connection with your testing are PT and INR.

PT stands for Prothrombin time test sometimes shortened to **protime.**

This is the name of the blood test used to measure the time it takes for your blood to clot.

INR stands for International Normalized Ratio

This is how the results of the PT test are reported and is the standardized way of stating the PT value. This standardization means that your results can be compared no matter which laboratory or hospital has run the tests.

It is important to become familiar with the term **INR**, and to understand the part this **number** plays in the **management** of your Coumadin levels. In simple terms,

If the **INR is too low** - blood clots cannot be prevented

If the **INR is too high** - there is an increased risk of bleeding

This is why it is important to have tests done **regularly** to ensure that the amount of Coumadin you are taking is sufficient to keep your INR number at the desired level. If your blood test shows that your INR number has increased or decreased your Coumadin dose may need to be adjusted. This is why your **dosage can change** from time to time.

Your Therapeutic Range

Your doctor, or anticoagulant specialist, will decide on the correct **target INR** for you and will aim to keep your INR number within a desired range. This is known as your Therapeutic Range, sometimes also referred to as Therapeutic Window.

People who do not use anticoagulant drugs will normally have an INR of 1 – this being the **normal rate** at which blood clots. Generally, the Therapeutic Range for a person who is at a higher risk of clotting will be set at an **INR of 2-3** – this means that their **blood will clot two to three times slower**.

Depending on your individual health circumstances, and why you have been prescribed Coumadin, your Therapeutic Range may be set **higher** or **lower** than this. It may also change from time to time according to your needs.

My Therapeutic Range was originally set at 2-3, however, after meeting with the consultants at London Bridge Hospital, who specialize in APS, ***my target INR*** *was set at 3-4. This seems to be the preferred range for those diagnosed with Hughes or antiphospholipid syndrome. Through time I have found that I tend to feel better when my INR is around 3 - 3.5 so after discussion with my local doctor my Therapeutic Range has been agreed at 2.5 - 3.5. This means my blood will take*

2½ to 3½ times longer to clot than someone who is not taking anticoagulant drugs.

Your doctor, or anticoagulant specialist, will monitor your INR using the blood test results and aim to keep you within your Therapeutic Range. Keeping in the target range will also reduce the risks of any **side effects.**

This diagram emphasizes the importance of keeping your INR within the Therapeutic Range that has been set for you.

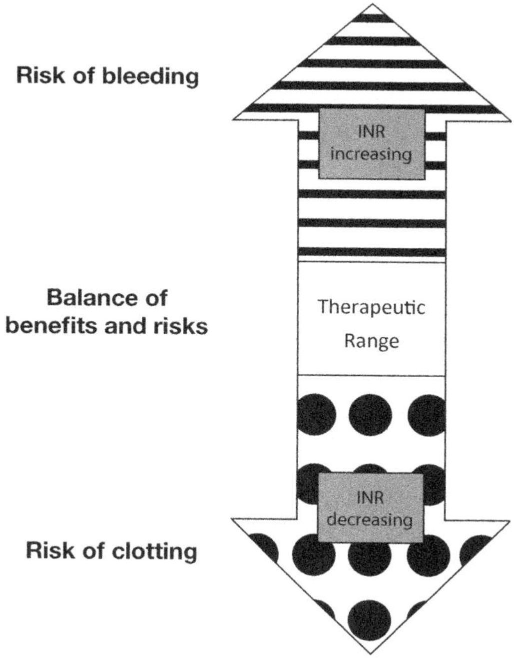

Your doctor will discuss what **'too high'** and **'too low'** is for you and if your INR levels go beyond these limits they will decide on an appropriate course of action to bring it back within your Therapeutic Range. This will depend on your individual circumstances but could include,

- remaining on the same dose of Coumadin but having more frequent blood tests (e.g. weekly) to monitor your INR
- adjusting your Coumadin dosage
- receiving 'blood thinning' injections, such as Heparin (or Fragmin), in addition to your Coumadin dosage until your INR returns to the desired range.

You should always know what your target INR and Coumadin dosage are and keep a record of these. When someone is first prescribed Coumadin they are generally issued with a booklet to record all the important information relating to their anticoagulation treatment - contacts, details of treatment, information required in an **emergency** and **details** such as the nature of your **underlying condition**. You can also use this booklet to record your daily dose and check off each dose after you have taken it.

*I carry my current booklet with me in a pouch along with all my medication. I also have an **SOS Talisman™ medical bracelet** which I wear at all times. This contains all my emergency information. There are many different types of medical alert devices available, even some smartphone apps, so you should be able to find one to suit your lifestyle!*

A lot of what you will read about Coumadin relates to the different factors that can affect how it performs and the dangers associated with this.

I was keen to understand more about this but the **biggest problem** I found was that the terminology used to explain these risks varied from one article to another and it could all get a bit confusing. **Anticoagulant effect, INR level, effectiveness of Coumadin** and **clot risk** are just some of the terms that are used to describe the workings of this complex drug.

I just wanted to be able to tell at a glance if something could put me **at risk of either bleeding or clotting!**

While these explanations are important, and, yes, I admit I have used much of this terminology too, *I wanted this book to be as straightforward and easy to understand as possible.*

In the chapters that follow, I have introduced a unique system called BloodWATCH which provides a quick key to the potential risk associated with any factor being discussed.

Anything which can put you at **increased risk of bleeding** will be denoted by *this text* or the following symbol:

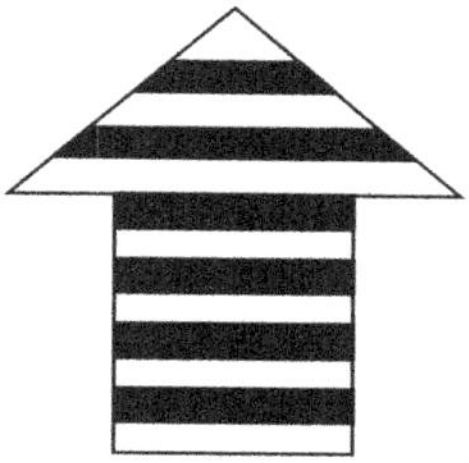

Anything which can put you at **increased risk of clotting** will be denoted by **this text** or the following symbol:

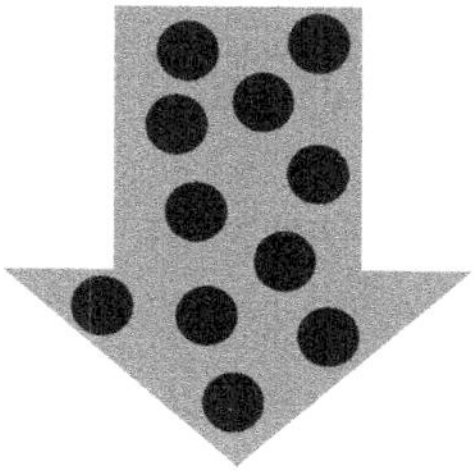

To link the BloodWATCH System with the other terminology used in this book I have put together a table which you can use as a quick reference. This should also assist you to interpret what you read about Coumadin elsewhere.

Increase in **anticoagulant effect**	Increased risk of bleeding	↑
Decrease in **anticoagulant effect**	Increased risk of clotting	↓
Increase in **'blood thinning'**	Increased risk of bleeding	↑
Decrease in **'blood thinning'**	Increased risk of clotting	↓
Increase in **clotting rate**	Increased risk of clotting	↓
Decrease in **clotting rate**	Increased risk of bleeding	↑
INR **below** Therapeutic Range	Increased risk of clotting	↓
INR **above** Therapeutic Range	Increased risk of bleeding	↑
Increase in **effect of Coumadin**	Increased risk of bleeding	↑
Decrease in **effect of Coumadin**	Increased risk of clotting	↓
Increasing **INR**	Increased risk of bleeding	↑
Decreasing **INR**	Increased risk of clotting	↓
Reduced platelet function	Increased risk of bleeding	↑

For more information on BloodWATCH or to download a copy of this table visit **www.eatonwarfarin.com**

CHAPTER 6

Vitamin K and Coumadin: what you need to know

One of the reasons that monitoring of your INR is so critical is that the performance of Coumadin can alter considerably when it interacts with other substances. One thing that can have a **significant influence on Coumadin,** and affect your INR, is **Vitamin K.**

As we discussed in section 2, the **clotting factors depend on Vitamin K** to do their job. This means that the amount of Vitamin K available in your body will affect how quickly the blood clots.

The body only stores very small amounts of Vitamin K so the big factor here is the amount of Vitamin K that you eat.

The **key** for people who are taking Coumadin is to try and eat approximately the same amount of Vitamin K, each week. Trying to be **consistent** and eating similar amounts each week will help to keep your INR fairly stable and within your therapeutic range. Most importantly, you want to **avoid big or sudden changes** in the amount of Vitamin K in your diet.

An **increased amount of Vitamin K** can **lower your INR** making Coumadin **less effective** and potentially increasing the risk of blood clots.

A *decreased amount of Vitamin K* can **increase your INR** making Coumadin **more effective** and putting you at risk of bleeding.

Just as importantly, you should not consider eliminating Vitamin K from your diet because you are concerned about it affecting your INR.

The key is to make only small changes and ensure consistency.

What foods contain Vitamin K?

Only a small number of foods contain **Vitamin K** in large quantities. The main foods that have a **high Vitamin K content** are dark green leafy vegetables such as **spinach**, **kale** and **beet greens** and oils such as **canola** and **olive oil**.

Other foods which contain Vitamin K but in much smaller amounts include dairy products, eggs, milk, fruit, liver and potatoes.

Vitamin K can also be found in **substantial amounts** in many processed and fast foods. This is because a lot of these foods are being cooked in, or produced using, Vitamin K rich oils. Some of the food groups where this has been detected include **burgers, potato chips, fast food fries, salad dressings** and even **cakes** although the actual Vitamin K content can vary greatly from brand to brand.

I have always loved eating salads and, growing up, I was always told how important it was to ***'eat your greens'.*** *I also used to eat a lot of* ***'super foods'*** *such as spinach, raw broccoli, wheatgrass and spirulina. Since I have been taking Coumadin I have found I have had to reduce my consumption of vitamin K rich foods, particularly broccoli and spinach. I also try to make sure I eat the same amounts of these foods each week. I don't calculate my* ***Vitamin K*** *level precisely each day but I have got to know the Vitamin K content of my favorite foods and I have learnt to judge the quantities I require. For instance, I now know that a single cup of spinach can contain dramatically more Vitamin K than a whole iceberg lettuce!*

Vitamin K Content of Common Foods

All foods can be categorized by the number of **micrograms** of Vitamin K they contain in a **100g serving.**

LOW - less than 20 micrograms
– these foods do not contain enough Vitamin K to have any significant impact.

MEDIUM - 20 to 80 micrograms
– count these foods as part of your daily Vitamin K intake.

HIGH - over 80 micrograms
– take care with these foods and make sure your intake is consistent. Too much of these could significantly decrease your INR and put you at risk of clotting.

The following table gives the vitamin K content and category of some everyday foods. For a more comprehensive list of foods, go to www.eatonwarfarin.com.

***Remember**, you do not have to completely avoid eating foods containing Vitamin K. It is more important to limit your intake and **eat roughly the same amount each day** – avoid having no Vitamin K one day and a large amount the next!*

	What does a 100g serving look like? ◊◊	Amount of Vitamin K per 100g (mcg) ◊	Category
Fruit + Veg			
Apple, Granny S.	1 small	3.2	**LOW**
Asparagus, boiled	7 spears	50.6	**MED**
Avocado ◊◊◊	½ small	21	**MED**
Banana ◊◊◊	1 small	0.5	**LOW**
Beet greens	2½ cups	400	**HIGH**
Blueberries, raw	⅔ cup	20	**MED**
Broccoli, raw	1 cup chopped	101.6	**HIGH**
Brussels sprouts	5 sprouts	177	**HIGH**
Carrot, boiled	⅔ cup	13.7	**LOW**
Endive, raw	2 cups chopped	231	**HIGH**
Grapes, raw	1 cup	14.6	**LOW**
Grapefruit ◊◊◊◊	½ medium	< 0.01	**LOW**
Iceberg lettuce	1½ cups shredded	24.1	**MED**
Kale, raw leaf	¾ cup	705	**HIGH**
Kohlrabi, boiled	¾ cup	0.1	**LOW**
Parsley, raw leaf	1½ cups	1640	**HIGH**
Peas, boiled	⅔ cup	26	**MED**
Potato, baked	½ medium	2	**LOW**

	What does a 100g serving look like? ◊◊	Amount of Vitamin K per 100g (mcg) ◊	Category
Fruit + Veg			
Radicchio, raw	2½ cups shredded	255	**HIGH**
Spinach, raw	3 cups	483	**HIGH**
Oils + Fats			
Butter	6 tbsp.	4.8	**LOW**
Canola oil	7 tbsp.	71.3	**MED**
Coconut oil	7 tbsp.	0.5	**LOW**
Margarine	7 tbsp.	92	**HIGH**
Olive oil	7 tbsp.	60.2	**MED**
Peanut oil	7 tbsp.	0.7	**LOW**
Sesame oil	7 tbsp.	13.6	**LOW**
Soybean oil	7 tbsp.	184	**HIGH**
Sunflower oil	7 tbsp.	5.4	**LOW**
Other			
Beef, roast	3 slices	1.4	**LOW**
Cheese, cheddar	small cup grated	2.9	**LOW**
Chicken, breast	1 small fillet	0.3	**LOW**
Coffee, instant	3½ fl.oz	1.9	**LOW**
Eggs, raw ◊◊◊◊◊	2 large	7	**LOW**

	What does a 100g serving look like? ◊◊	Amount of Vitamin K per 100g (mcg) ◊	Category
Other			
Hash Brown, fried	⅔ cup	20	**MED**
Mayonnaise	7 tbsp.	25	**MED**
Milk, whole	3½ fl.oz	0.3	**LOW**
Water	3½ fl.oz	< 0.01	**LOW**
Yogurt, low fat plain	⅘ of a pot	0.2	**LOW**

◊ these values have been sourced from the USDA Nutrient Database for Standard Reference Release 27.

◊◊ these serving sizes are provided as a guide only. The amount contained in these servings could vary depending on your interpretation of the sizes and factors such as how finely you chop your vegetables or how much you can squash in a cup! If you need precise 100g servings you should weigh or measure the portions yourself!

◊◊◊ these foods might be low in Vitamin K but have high potassium levels

◊◊◊◊ while low in Vitamin K, grapefruit has been reported to interact with Coumadin – see chapter 7

◊◊◊◊◊ the Vitamin K content given for eggs is Vitamin K2. All other values quoted are Vitamin K1.

For more advice on portion sizes and daily Vitamin K intake visit
www.eatonwarfarin.com

CHAPTER 7

Other interactions with Coumadin

There are many other factors that can affect your Coumadin therapy and make managing your INR more difficult.

So many substances can interact with Coumadin - food, medication, dietary supplements to name but a few! Add to that other factors, such as hydration and how differently individuals can respond to Coumadin, and you can see how things can get complicated!

It is good, therefore, to **have an awareness** of how **different factors** can affect the way Coumadin works and how these, in turn, could significantly put you at risk.

Other Medication

Coumadin is *particularly susceptible to interaction with other medication.*

Problems are least likely to occur with medication that you have been on long term and take regularly. When your initial Coumadin dosage is calculated any other regular medication that you already take will be reflected in the level of Coumadin you are prescribed.

Complications are more likely with medication that is taken in the **short term** such as antibiotics or painkillers as these can cause more sudden interactions with your Coumadin therapy.

One particular type of medication which should be treated with extra caution is the group of medicines known as **Non-steroidal anti-inflammatory drugs (NSAIDs)** as they can significantly increase the **risk of bleeding** without any corresponding change in INR.

Some examples[1] of the medications which may interact with Coumadin include,

Increased risk of bleeding 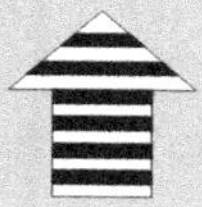	**Increased risk of clotting** 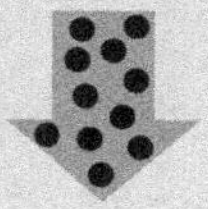
Nonsteroidal anti-inflammatories e.g. *aspirin* *ibuprofen* *diclofenac*	Cold/cough remedies containing zinc e.g. **zinc lozenges** **zinc sulfate syrup**

[1]This is not a complete list of the medications which may interact with Coumadin. For more information on possible interactions visit www.eatonwarfarin.com

Increased risk of bleeding	**Increased risk of clotting**
Cox-2 Inhibitors e.g. *celecoxib*	Laxatives e.g. **Senokot®**
Certain groups of Antibiotics e.g. *penicillins* *tetracyclines* *erythromycins*	Epilepsy medication e.g. **primidone** **phenytoin** **carbamzepine**
Cold/flu remedies e.g. containing *aspirin*	Oral Contraceptives e.g. **Microgynon®** **Cilest®**
SSRI Antidepressants e.g. *fluoxetine* *citalopram*	
Antifungals e.g. *fluconazole* *ketoconazole*	

Remember - any medication could potentially interact with Coumadin, or affect the way your body responds to Coumadin. Therefore, do not stop or start any new treatment without first discussing this fully with your doctor.

Foods, Herbs and Supplements

Additionally, there are a considerable number of foods, herbs and dietary supplements which have been reported to affect how Coumadin performs.

As a **quick reference** I have listed some of the more significant, or commonly reported interactions which should be **avoided** or **taken with care**.

		RISK
Chamomile	increases the effect of Coumadin	↑
Coenzyme Q10	structurally related to Vitamin K	↓
Cranberry Juice	HIGH risk of bleeding – avoid drinking	↑
Dong quai	significant increase in risk of bleeding	↑
Garlic	medicinal garlic can increase blood thinning	↑

		RISK
Ginger	connected with reports of abnormal bleeding	↑
Ginkgo	connected with reports of abnormal bleeding	↑
Grapefruit Juice	inhibits metabolism of Coumadin - avoid	↑
Green Tea	large volumes may increase risk of clots	↓
Licorice root	increases the effect of Coumadin	↑
Mango	increased risk of bleeding – limit consumption	↑
Menthol	may decrease the effect of Coumadin	↓
Protein	high protein diets linked to decrease in INR	↓
St John's Wort	reduces the effect of Coumadin	↓
Vitamin C	high doses may reduce the effect of Coumadin	↓
Vitamin E	may increase the INR at high doses	↑
Willow bark	has properties similar to Aspirin	↑

This is not an exhaustive list. For more information on interactions with Coumadin visit www.eatonwarfarin.com

Other Factors

Alcohol

Excessive use of alcohol, **particularly binge drinking**, can lead to an increase in INR and a higher risk of bleeding. Studies do not suggest, however, that you need to avoid alcohol altogether if you are taking Coumadin. General advice is not to exceed 2 units of alcohol in a day and that having a small amount to drink regularly is preferable to drinking larger quantities occasionally. The key, as with so many other things for Coumadin users, is moderation and consistency!

Tobacco

Studies on the effects of smoking on Coumadin are a little inconclusive but there is a general consensus that some of the chemicals in tobacco have the effect of decreasing Coumadin levels in the body which could lead to a decrease in INR. It is generally found, therefore, that smokers require a higher dosage of Coumadin to maintain their correct INR levels than if they didn't smoke. However, the biggest concern would be *if a smoker stopped using tobacco products suddenly* as this could result in a sharp increase in INR and high risk of bleeding.

Illness 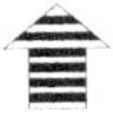 or 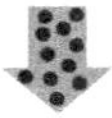

Common illnesses, such as colds, flu, vomiting or diarrhea, can alter your metabolism and affect how your body handles Coumadin. Any upset in absorption from the gut, or loss of fluids, can change the levels of Coumadin in your blood dramatically. If you are unwell you should always try and get your INR tested as early as possible to monitor any changes that may have taken place.

Although my INR generally remains quite stable, I have had a number of episodes when there have been big fluctuations in my INR levels. These have been due to factors such as a ***change in diet*** *or taking* ***other medication.***

One incident was when I needed to take ***painkillers****. The painkillers interacted with my Coumadin,* ***causing my INR to increase****. Now, when I feel I need to take painkillers, I communicate with my doctor so that he can keep an eye on my INR levels.*

A more worrying episode was when I decided I wanted to lose some weight and tried to change my diet. I specifically wanted to reduce my intake of sugars, processed foods and refined carbohydrates. I was careful with the amount of green leafy vegetables I was eating, trying to be ***consistent,*** *as I was aware of the effect that too much* ***Vitamin K*** *could have on* ***decreasing the effect of Coumadin****. However, I forgot that* ***protein intake*** *could* ***also affect Coumadin*** *and as a result of my new diet my* ***protein levels increased****. I started to lack energy and had problems focusing my eyes which at first I just put down to being tired. However, I ended up feeling exhausted and wanting to sleep all the time. Eventually when it got to the stage that I even lacked the energy to talk or to make sense of things I made an appointment to have my INR checked. My range at the time was meant to be between 2.5 and 3.5 - my results came back as 1.6! As a result, I was given an* ***extra 1mg*** *of Coumadin* ***every 3 days*** *until my INR returned to its* ***normal range*** *and* ***settled.***

Through experiencing these episodes, I have come to be able to recognize when my INR falls below, or goes above, my therapeutic range. During periods when my INR has fluctuated, I have recorded the symptoms and feelings I have had. As a result, I have become better at ***recognizing the symptoms more quickly*** *so that whenever any of these early warning signals occur I can go to my doctor and request an INR test. Where the warning symptoms are only slight I am becoming* *more able to counterbalance changes to my INR by making small adjustments to my diet.*

Please remember that we are all individuals and that other people may experience **no symptoms** or **completely different symptoms** when their INR levels are too high, or too low.

What is **important** is to,

- be aware of the factors that could potentially affect your INR levels
- **learn** to recognize any early warning signals that could indicate there may be a change in **your** INR
- request an INR test if you are concerned about symptoms so that any **changes can be caught early.**

You may find it useful to record any symptoms or feelings you experience when you have a low INR, or high INR. This can help you to become familiar with any early signs you should look out for that could point to a change in your INR levels. If you want to do this for yourself, a sample of my symptoms record can be found at the website below.

CHAPTER 8

Alternatives to Coumadin

There are a number of alternatives to Coumadin starting to become available, and more new drugs are likely to be developed in the future. It is hoped that the new breed of drugs will be easier to manage, having less interactions with food and other medications, but there is still a long way to go before these are a suitable option for everyone requiring an anticoagulant.

Currently, Coumadin continues to be the medication of choice for most case scenarios and, for people managing well on Coumadin, and whose INR is stable, there would be **little benefit** to changing to a different medicine. Where there are other reasons why Coumadin is not suitable, you may be prescribed something else.

Other anticoagulants you may come across include:

- dabigatran (Pradaxa®)
- rivaroxaban (Xarelto®)
- enoxaparin (Clexane®)
- heparin injections (such as Fragmin®)

Dabigatran and rivaroxaban are similar to Coumadin in that **the main risk factor** when taking these is **bleeding**.

However, there are a couple of distinct differences between Coumadin and dabigatran and rivaroxaban.

1. There is no test to monitor the effect of these drugs on blood clotting in the way that the INR blood test monitors the effect of Coumadin.

2. There is **no specific antidote** to dabigatran and rivaroxaban to stop bleeding quickly in the way that a **vitamin K injection** can **reverse the effects of Coumadin.**

The pros and cons of any alternatives should be discussed with your doctor, or anticoagulant specialist. You should not stop taking Coumadin unless instructed to do so as you may **risk developing blood clots** or **having a stroke**.

I talked to my doctor about whether any of the alternatives to Coumadin would be suitable for me.

The doctor explained that many of the alternatives have still to go through full clinical testing; some have passed trials for venous clots only. As I am at risk of arterial clots none of the alternative medications are available to me yet and Coumadin continues to be the most suitable medication for my condition.

CHAPTER 9

In Summary: Managing your Coumadin safely

Dietary Do's and Don'ts

Managing your Coumadin therapy and INR levels can be a bit of a balancing act. We have seen that one of the biggest keys to getting this right is careful management of your body's intake of food, drink and other substances.

To summarize:

DO

- Keep your diet consistent
- Eat similar types of food and portion sizes from week to week
- Be aware of foods that can interact with Coumadin
- Eat consistent amounts of green leafy vegetables and any other foods with a high/medium Vitamin K content
- Get your INR checked if changes to your diet have occurred
- Understand the levels of vitamin K and protein contained within the foods you like to eat. Keep your consumption of these consistent.
- Maintain good hydration

- Limit your alcohol intake
- Avoid smoking or tobacco products

DON'T

- Make drastic changes to your diet
- Stop smoking suddenly
- Go on crash diets, protein based diets or fast long term
- Take over the counter medication, such as aspirin or ibuprofen, without consulting your doctor
- Take new medicines or supplements without discussing with your doctor
- Eliminate foods containing Vitamin K from your diet completely
- Make sudden changes in the amount of protein you are eating
- Allow yourself to become dehydrated
- Binge drink or consume excessive quantities of alcohol

Reducing Risks

To further reduce any of the risks of being a Coumadin patient, try and stick to these simple guidelines:

- Take your medication exactly as it was prescribed i.e. your correct dose at the same time each day.
- Carefully read the information leaflet that comes with your medication.
- If you miss a dose OR take too much, **FOLLOW THE DIRECTIONS ON THE LEAFLET IN THE MEDICATION BOX.**
- Be aware of side effects and warning signs. If you detect any of these, speak to your doctor immediately.
- Set an alarm to remind you to take your medication, and record doses taken.
- Set up reminders to **re-order your prescriptions. Never run out.**
- **Check** you do not have any conditions or medical reasons why you should not be on Coumadin, including pregnancy; discuss all the issues with your doctor.

- Don't miss your INR test appointments.
- If you have any signs or symptoms of bleeding contact your doctor immediately.
- Never self-dose unless you have agreed this with your doctor or anticoagulant specialist.
- Use a softer toothbrush to reduce gum bleeding and visit your dentist regularly to maintain tooth and gum health.
- If you need dental treatment, or any surgical procedure, discuss your condition thoroughly with your dentist/doctor beforehand.
- Wear a medical alert item containing all your health and emergency information and/or use a medical alert smartphone app.
- Carry your anticoagulation record book with you at all times.
- Keep a good first aid kit containing some wound dressing pads in your car. Also try and carry a couple of wound dressing pads and plasters with you in a pouch or handbag.

- If you have been involved in an emergency situation and require urgent medical help, try and ensure all those dealing with you are aware that you are on Coumadin or blood thinning medication.

- Avoid contact sports or hazardous activities that may result in cuts, bruises or broken bones.

- Take extra care when carrying out tasks and repairs around the house. Do what you can to minimize falls and cuts, such as moving items that may cause you to trip or being careful when climbing ladders.

- If you become pregnant, speak to your doctor immediately about an alternative to Coumadin during pregnancy.

I hope the information in this book has been useful to you. The aim of this book was to present a basic overview of the implications of taking Coumadin as well as a synopsis of my own experiences. As mentioned previously, I am not a medical practitioner and I do not have any medical training, so please consult your doctor about any medical issue you may have.

If you wish to comment or discuss any of the points mentioned in this book, please visit our website.

List of Resources Used

Leaflet insert from Coumadin medication

www.nhs.uk

www.nps.org.au NPS Medicinewise

www.anticoagulation.com.au

www.ptinr.com

McCance and Widdowson's The Composition of Foods 7th Summary Edition, 2014

USDA Nutrient Database for Standard Reference Release 27

The Coumadin (Warfarin) Help Book – Diana M Schneider

Nutescu EA, Shapiro NL, Ibrahim S, West P – Coumadin and its interactions with foods, herbs and other dietary supplements. Expert Opin. Drug Saf. (2006) 5(3):433-451

Biss TT, Adamson AJ, Seal CJ, Kamali F (2011). The potential impact of dietary vitamin K status on anticoagulation control in children receiving Coumadin. Paediatric Haematology & Oncology, 28(5), 425-427. doi:10.3109/08880018.2011.562276

Conger K (2010). Slow on the uptake. Stanford Medicine, 27(3), 46.

Goldhaber SZ, Fiumara K. Cardiology Patient Page. A patient's guide to taking Coumadin/Coumadin. Retrieved from http://circ.ahajournals.org/content/119/8/e220.full. Circulation 2009; 119: e220-e222doi:10.1161/CIRCULATION.108.803957.

Useful Links

American Heart Association

www.heart.org/HEARTORG/

American Lung Association

www.lung.org/

American Stroke Association

www.strokeassociation.org/STROKEORG/

Arrhythmia Alliance

www.aa-international.org

Atrial Fibrillation Association

www.atrialfibrillation-us.org

Hughes Syndrome Foundation

www.hughes-syndrome.org

International Society on Thrombosis and Haemostasis

www.isth.org

National Stroke Association

www.stroke.org

Index

Made in the USA
Monee, IL
04 November 2026

67378957R00046